I0406613

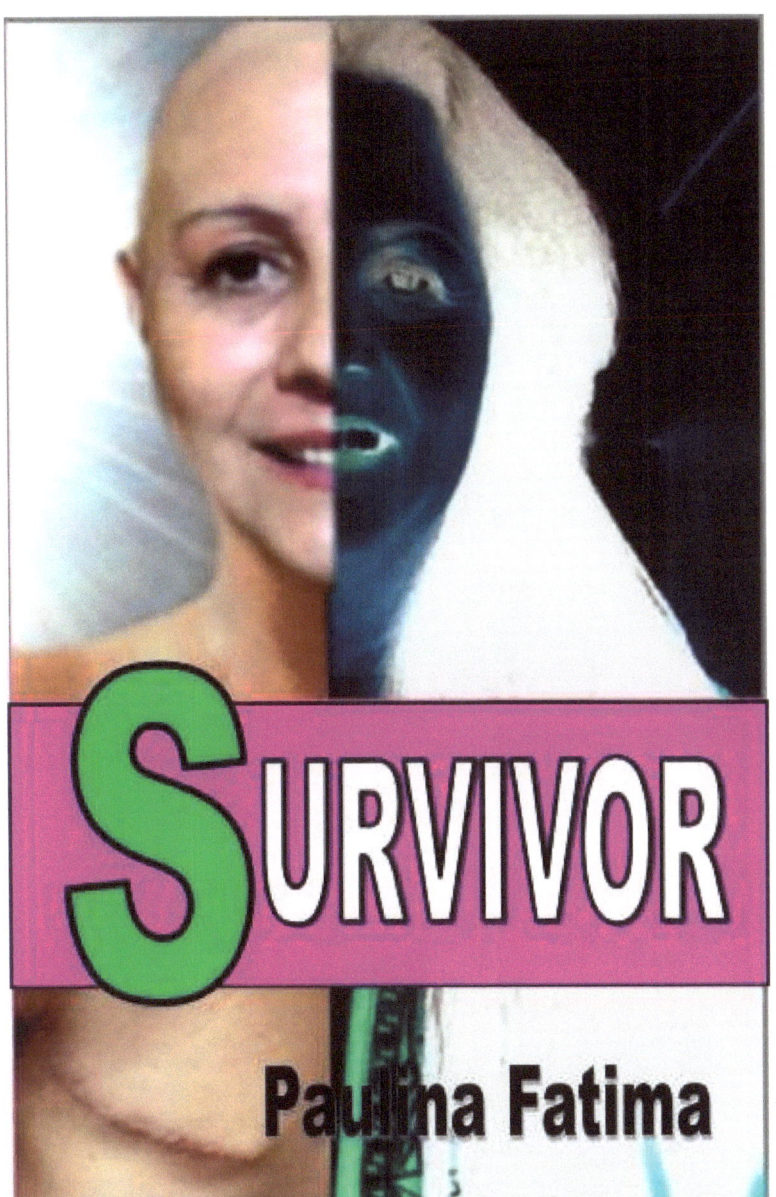

UNUSUAL DEDICATION

I especially dedicate this book to my husband Ramadan and to my girl Atiat. They both have been here, very close, getting me up when I was without strength, making me smile when my eyes bags were deeply touching my soul. They were feeding me when I just could flavor their love from their hugs.

I also dedicate this book to my other children Glauco and Roberto, to my daughters in law Tefy and Ester. Every one of them cheered me up and advised me at their way. Tefy was with me at the toughest moment on that first appointment with the oncologist; I will never forget her supporting words.

My son Roberto was persistent and pending on my advance, demanding more from me, because he needs to recover his fighter mother. Glauquito, my oldest son and his wife Ester from the other side of the continent, were connected to me for endless hours by skype in actual time. To my son's parents in law, Janet and Javier, to Norma, the grandmother from Uruguay and to my other son's mother in law Remedios in Spain.

To my mother, (R.I.P.), who was in Cuba without knowing my terrible moment but suspecting that something happened around. She knew it at the end.

To my brother Paco and my sister in law Tania who knew what was going on but they couldn't say anything to my mother.

To my friend who is also my soul sister, Gloria Bolaños, who convinced me that is possible to touch the sky with our hands if we have FAITH, she called me up three or four times each day during eight months and she is still here with me.

To my friend Rolando Baute, always faithful. His cards told me all that happened six months in advance.

To my friend Juan José, who was supporting me, he was so cute.

To my friends Vilma and Alberto Planas who kept me in their prayers. To my friend Vicky Roig.

To my unconditional friend Ricardo Belmont for his affection, his economical support and his daily concerning. To Giova and Guido who didn't let that I wasn´t without my natural medicines from Perú.

To my friend Juan Carlos who helped me greatly in writing this book.

To **"La Diosa del Flow"**, Felix, Nene, Omar and Adarin. I adore them because they always helped me and love me.

To all of those who were anyway supporting me in the anonymity, all my **Facebook** friends, hundreds of people who I don't know personally but who follow my story on the web every day, cheering me up to go on fighting.

Thanks to all of you.

Paulina Fatima.

YOU WILL SURVIVE

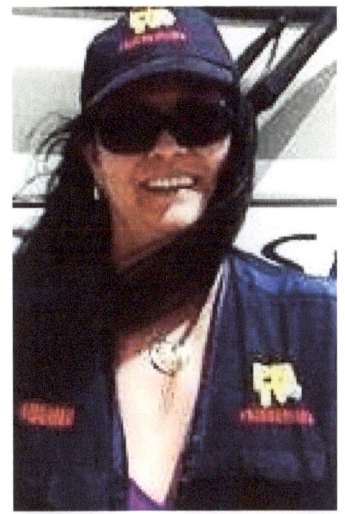

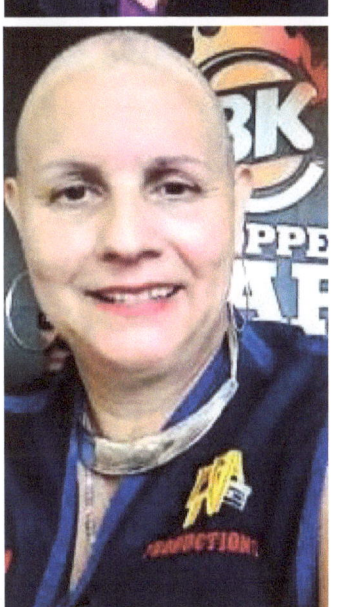

You will Survive,

Yes, You Can

To you who have begun reading this book, thank you.

I will Survive is the first of a campaign that begins with this Volume I, "*Yes you Can*".

Each volume carries a message of hope and I will show you tools to prevent, combat and live with dignity during this process.

This first book begins a process of getting to know each other. In it, I open my heart to you and capture on paper a number of strong feelings, medical investigations and experiences that have filled my life in the last few years.

You will also view pictures, read short stories, and enjoy or hate them. I wrote these during different times of my life, and I relived them like a movie, in each chemo therapy session at wonderful Jackson Memorial Hospital as I sat for hours in a comfortable recliner waiting for my session to end.

I hope that reading this book and the rest of the collection, will be an inspiration to continue and I envision a better life for each person that reads it.

GREATER KNOWLEDGE OF THE SUFFERING MAKES US HAVE ABSOLUTE CONTROL OF THE SITUATION

It's necessary to get enthused and follow the advice here suggested, meals and attitude in life, so that you can build on what you have learned to be able to live a better and more coherent life. I too have learned of other people and learn more each and every day.

- Have faith in God
- Away from your life the disagreement.
- Away the resentment
- Remove the hate of its life
- Act straight ahead and be combative
- Be informed about your medical condition
- Learn about your immune system
- Be a positive person

We need to act to combat this terrible illness and we must be well informed in order to do so. Our immunological system is our protector, ready to defend us, but unfortunately many people have no idea of what the immunological system is and that is serious.

Dear friends, at 50, I have learned the complexity and cruelty of many people. Even though it sounds incredible, I look back on my history and realize that my learning experience was very slow during my first 50 years.

The level of naiveté and thinking that all people are good and love us is actually ridiculous. That doesn't exist, you that are reading me, please place your feet firmly on the ground and begin to pander to yourself because nobody else will do it for you. I can assure you. I also have to recognize that there are great families that nurture their members. But whatever your situation, don't falter and trust, the human being is designed to utilize his sense of inspiration and psyche to rise above adversity and be a fighter for your life. It's in your hands to take stock of it. Nothing is more important and stronger than the power of the mind and our spirit, but not only to conquer cancer but to face life.

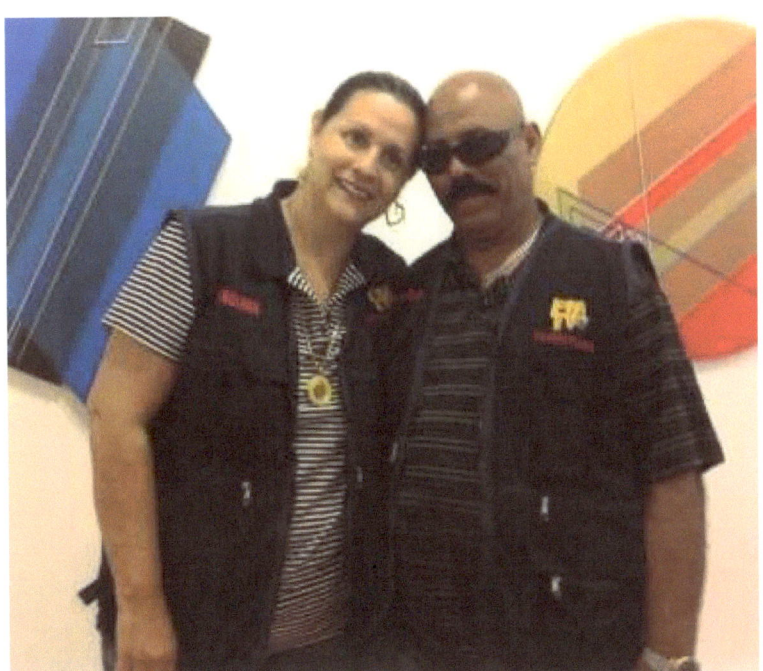

This photo corresponds to the day in which they said to me that it had cancer.

WHO IS PAULINA FATIMA?

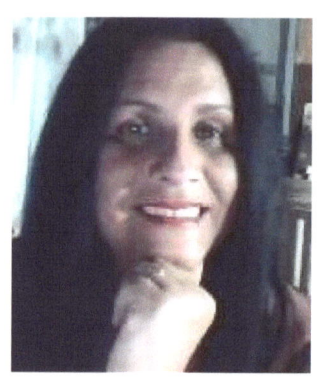

My name is Paulina Fatima Gonzalez Gonzalez. I was born in La Habana, on June 8th, 1960, and now I am better known as Paulina Aly because of my husband's last name who is Ramadan Aly. I like helping people to find their dreams´ path. I love music, poetry and life, I love my family, my friends. I am very sentimental and I consider it as a failure of my personality which I should change that is what my friend Gloria always says to me.

I studied 3 years of chemistry engineering at CUJAE. I was a writer for the Cuban television, a scriptwriter of a soap opera called *"**Enamorada**"*, whose adviser was the maestro Eliseo Altunaga and Mrs. Venegas. Also I was a writer for children programs at channel 6 such as "*Don Mínimo*" "*Había una vez*" and many others initiatives on television and on the literary world. This is only some things I have done in Cuba. After, I got out of Cuba and I went to Europe for 7 years where thousands of things occurred and are counted in another book called "*Historias de una cubana emigrante*", these experiences have helped for being the woman I am. I came to United States in 2002 and I have traveled to Perú in big projects and responsibilities.

My performance in life can be summarized as a woman who doesn't give up, who has fought and will continue fighting for a better world, not only for her but for everybody around her, too.

Since I left Cuba, I have traveled the world, I have known different cultures and I have had either positive experiences or forced ones; I have enjoyed the luxury of a presidential suite, a cabin on an American Marine ship at the Mediterranean Sea, as well as I have slept in hostile places. I lived in a small hostel when I arrived to Spain, coexisting with witches, prostitutes, drug consumers, drug dealers, but without bending my way. I have known how to bright among the unknown of the underworld in my first years of exile. I have known the hunger, the loneliness, the betrayal, the forced distance from the loved ones. I have been offered since the most severe vices until the oldest professions for surviving, however, in those chaotic moments, I have been able to continue without losing my dignity, not doing anything that I could be regretted for nowadays, because God has always been on my side and another option has always emerged.

I have been able to work on my way towards the horizon of my expectations as a human being and I have been able to go ahead and up based on my daily effort.

I also knew the other side of the coin of our Mother Nation, Spain, where nice people live who will be always in my heart, and who were very important in my life, like Julian Riego and Juan Carlos Fraile.

I, I am as I am, I am not perfect, I don´t intend to be perfect, I don´t like to be perfect, only God knows what this word really means, I am just a person who have taken all the little details from life, the beautiful ones and until the misfortune ones, as a raw material to reflect on every falling down and getting up for reemerging, without losing my smile and my wishes of living.

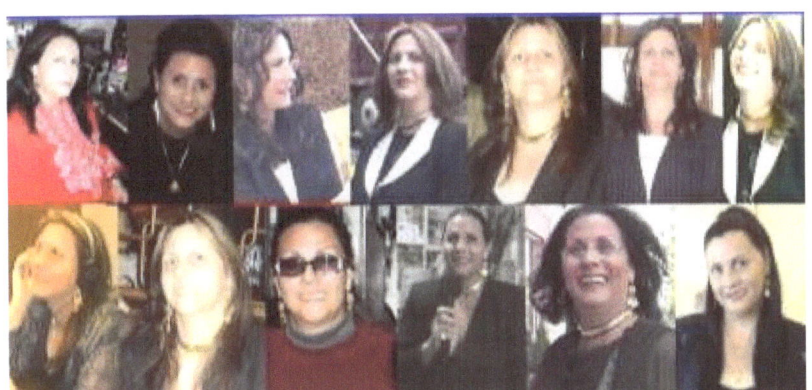

NOTHING IS ETERNAL, NOT EVEN THE DEEPEST PAIN

If we have a medical or spiritual situation and as a first option we lie down in bed to feel sorry about ourselves, to stay crying for days, to consume alcohol or drugs, the problem will be triple, because there will be the same situation with other subsequent problems derived from the mistaken reaction to the solution given to the problem.

When you experience a thought of complaining, reflect and take a second to look around you.

- Look at your neighbor, your workmate, what is happening to them
- Watch the news, see what is happening in faraway countries
- You have to be conscious that there are many people who don´t have anything of

the things you have and they survive every second in life

- That there are thousands of children who die each day in this world just because of lacking of food, without any option

- That your problem is not larger than the ones of many others

- Neither you nor I are the center of the universe, we are just a little dot inside a platform

- Look at the ones who don´t have one or two of their limbs like arms or hands and make an effort and drive a car

- Look at those who don´t have legs and enroll in a dancing contest showing to the world their spectacular prostheses

- Look at those who have terminal cancer and they stick to life for one more second.

I would like you are in this list of courageous people.
Have you ever thought of all of this?

However, you, who have almost everything, complain of any minor detail, you allow yourself of having **DEPRESSION** whatever the reason is.

Consider consciously my words and remember that:

- You have a job to do and a responsibility in this world
- You are important
- You are unique, there are not 2 like you
- The world needs you, that´s why you were created

MY 50 YEARS OLD. A GOOD STARTING POINT.

I celebrate my 50 years old with a great party, as my world had a new beginning, or maybe it was the beginning of the end. *"My friends"* and some members of the family came and I gave a strange speech where I almost said goodbye to life.

It was a highly organized party. Good food and drink, delicious desserts, where singers were dedicating songs to me. I wouldn´t wish to mention anybody, the ones who were there knew what happened, other didn´t come and just sent flowers and presents.

What an incredible thing! Two years later, due to excess of stress, a bad nutrition and many other details made me get sick and one day, I was told that I had cancer. The funniest part of the story was that most of my friends disappeared once they knew of my sickness.

The excuses started to show up, a lot of work, we don´t want to see you this way, we feel badly for the way you feel, it´s better for another occasion, relax, go to bed, we will see maybe next week, no, Pauli, I am busy, don´t worry, we´ll see you, we will see you tomorrow; That happened and hurt me but here I am, I have never lost my smile.

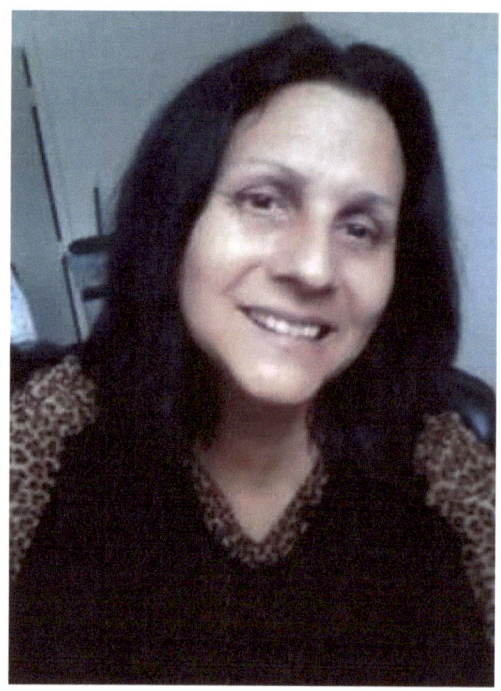

THE MOMENT OF TRUTH: THE FEAR

It is very hard when you go to the doctor's office for a routine check-up, for the yearly mammogram, and things get complicated. Overnight you become very important, but not because of your incredible talents, but rather because you are incredibly sick. You feel something strange is happening. The woman taking the mammogram images takes one, then another, she checks it, she comes near you, she tells you she'll be right back; we start again, raise your arm, she lifts your head, she presses harder, etc. etc. Then she leaves the room again and you are left alone with all your doubts and questions for over forty minutes. In fact, all the delay, all those images, absolutely everything indicates and lets you know that there's indeed a problem.

The situation becomes severe because you feel a fear that you never knew existed; a type of fear that is not described within the meaning of the word itself; it is something completely different. It's the type of fear that gives you a stomachache, a bellyache, you feel you want to urinate, you want to defecate, all together, you even want to vomit; all of that happens while you wait for them to tell you what is happening to you.

After those fateful forty minutes, they tell you to go in to see the doctor, she is waiting for you. I walked as fast as I could to the doctor's office, and there she was, a Philippine doctor, petite and plump and I sat next to her. She was reviewing my files, but, practically without looking up at me, she said coldly: *"we have found that you have a tumor. You have mass in your right breast."*

"It is very likely that you have cancer in your right breast, in the lower quadrant. Your mammogram shows a number five bitrates, so I'm afraid we'll have to do a biopsy and the whole routine process to know what stage your in.

In any case, there is always the possibility that it may be a benign mass; but I must let you know that based on the form in which it appears on the mammogram, we believe that it is a carcinoma; cancer; and that is all I can tell you for today. We'll go ahead now and make another appointment for you to do a biopsy. "

In the midst of all this, I was still in awe. My husband held my hand and I was trembling, I was cold and sweaty, the situation was complicated. Besides, I can't understand the coldness with which they can say something that is so serious for you, perhaps it is the best way, it is the procedure they use with all patients in the United States. I don't know how the story goes in other countries.

Finally, after a short while, she realized how badly I felt and said to me: *"But this is not the end of the world. You must realize that you are on time here in this office to confront this situation. Don't worry, there's a solution for everything."* I could not take being in that room for one more second I couldn't deal with that doctor. I got up and left. My husband ran behind me, and she ran after him telling him *"leave her, leave her, she will be fine, come and I will give you the appointment for the tests that follow and for the biopsy.*

I met with my husband a few minutes later in the hospital's lobby. I was sitting motionless. My chest ached intensely; my heart was beating at full speed. It was all real; *I HAD CANCER.*

The routine of relentless days to overcome the disease was about to begin. There should be a wiser and calmer way to break the news to a patient. I am not a doctor, but I know that they are used to breaking those kinds of news because of the hundreds of cases that pass by their office. But for each one of us the experience is unique, that is why I think that there should be a less impactful way of breaking the news.

THE DEPRESSION AS STRONG AS THE CANCER

The depression is considered as the pandemic of the modern society. Nowadays, it affects two millions of people worldwide and this is the way everything is, a mess.

There are too many people sick of sadness, who can start from severe traumas of life summing up the diverse frustrations that form a series of negative factors.

It is embarrassing and the solution to the problem is individual, millions of people would have to change how to afford their life.

A depressive state may constitute a risky factor for the beginning of the sickness. The people affected by a chronic depression since some years ago, are often sad and tired, and they may have a highly probability of developing a kind of cancer. On the other hand, the cancer can also cause a depression: many people who are developing the sickness suffer of depression after they are diagnosed with cancer.

It is fundamental not to allow that this depression evolve and it should be treated because it may prevent a favorable progress.

Have 5 minutes, close your eyes and make an introspection, it means, an internal inspection. Observe and examine your own ideas, thoughts and feelings. After, go slowly and pass to retrospection, it means, have a look and an observation towards a past time. After these two exercises, ask yourself: Who am I? According to the answered gotten, you can reorganize your present for carrying out a project of your future life.

There is much to do yet and everything is in your hands and in what you really order to your brain.

OVERCOME THE FEAR TO DEATH

The moment when you receive the diagnosis is shocking; you suffer the anguish of death in an instant, you think in what is going to come, in the sight from others, in their misbehavior, the fear of this sickness in others, the bad image of sick people.

The delicate moment is the beginning of the process, the way it is assimilated, the reaction of the drugs and even the environment of the hospital, the person who has cancer enters in a depression state. In this point, if we don´t know how to control themselves, there are less possibilities of surviving and more possibilities for not following the treatment.

My father died of cancer when I was 15, and it was a traumatic experience, he was 5 years enduring and suffering. I have never forgotten neither that time nor the day of his death.

We shouldn´t forget that the term cancer is associated with death, in spite of the numerous advances that have been done in recent years for its diagnosis, treatment and prevention. But certainly the number of diagnosis resulted every year has improved, indicating that anyone can suffer of any kind of cancer and the possibilities of suffering of cancer are bigger while people get older.

The possibility of dying, the fear of treatment, the pain or suffering, or the imminent changes in the relationships with the family, the spouse, or the friends, are things that affect greatly the behavior of a sick person generating upset and depressive feelings. We shouldn´t forget that the cancer changes completely the life of the patient, of his or her family, and his or her social and work environment.

We, who have received a cancer diagnosis experience different levels of anguish and emotional tension where we include basically the important aspects of the life as a sick person:

- ✓ Fear of death
- ✓ Interruption of plans of life
- ✓ Changes on the body image and self-esteem
- ✓ Changes in social functions and lifestyles
- ✓ Money and legal Worrying

Every one reacts about these aspects in different forms and some of us may not suffer of severe depression or anxiety. All depends on the attitude and the positive message that you send to the brain.

I remember when the social assistant at the hospital asked me *"Have you already done your last will?"*

And I felt frozen, and these thoughts were on my mind quickly: Sickness, chemotherapy, catheters, surgery and testament…OMG! I thought…this is the end, but it was not more than a disagreeable routine that they have in this country, as the same rude way they communicate your diagnosis.

But well, coming back to the subject, it was found that the people who takes care of a person who suffers of cancer experience more anxiety and depression than the people who are not in charge of the caring of the sick person, and also the children are affected when one of the parents has cancer and is depressed, the child is in panic, feeling disproportionally the fear of the parent.

One study on women´s breast cancer demonstrated that the children of depressed patients have more possibilities of suffering emotional and behavior problems, that´s why is so important the self-control.

There are many mistaken ideas about cancer and about how people afford it; for example:

The sadness and the affliction because of cancer or any other sickness are normal reactions against the crisis that a person has to face for what is coming. All sick people experience these reactions in a moment or in another. However, as sadness is a common thing, it is important to distinguish between the normal levels of it and the real depression.

An important part about the caring of the sickness patient is to recognize that the depression has to be treated. Some people may have more problems than others for accepting the diagnosis of cancer. The serious depression is not only being sad or discouraged. That's why I insist on a positive attitude and the respect for life in order to assume the difficult moments.

When a person has had a cancer and it has been overcome, the fear is centered in the reappearance of it. The periodical checkups help us to diminish this fear.

However, the ideal thing is to adopt a healthy lifestyle, try to reduce stress, have time with friends and family, involve in leisure activities, work out and definitely, simplify life.

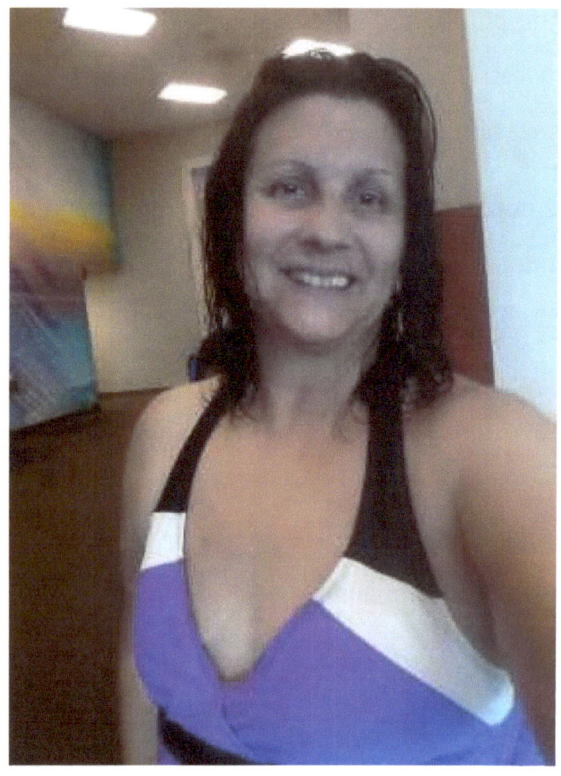

CATHETER AND PORT DAY ON MY CHEST

Asides from the biopsy, the insertion of the catheter has been the most traumatic procedure in my life. There are no words to describe the pain I felt on

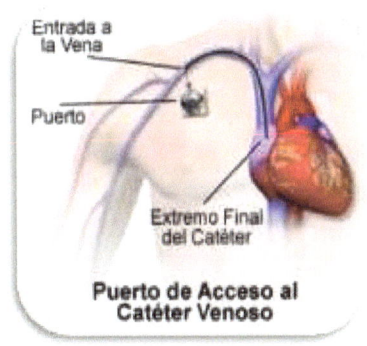

the day that I left the operating room when they inserted the catheter in me and the horrendous days that followed, one by one, for over nine months. I must also admit that not having problems with the arm veins, which I

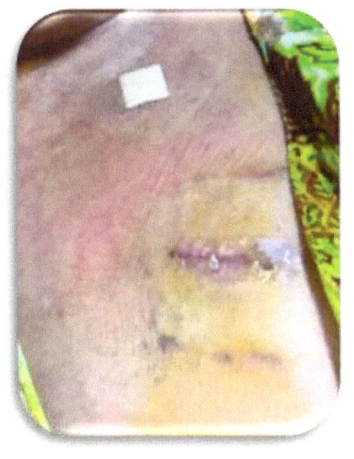

understand always get damaged, helps a lot to endure the long hours seated in the small cold chemotherapy room.

A catheter is a thin flexible tube inserted in a large vein in the body. It remains there as long as it needs to; in other words, until they know that you are well again. Mine was removed three months after the operation.

The catheter was attached to a port, which is a small round plastic or metal disc placed under the skin and which is used as a pump to control the speed in which the medication is administered in the catheter or port. An external pump remains outside the body; an internal pump is surgically placed just below the skin. I consider this procedure to be extremely painful, and even three years later, I feel terror chills in my stomach just remembering it.

CHEMOTHERAPY: A FATEFUL AND CONTROVERSIAL WORD

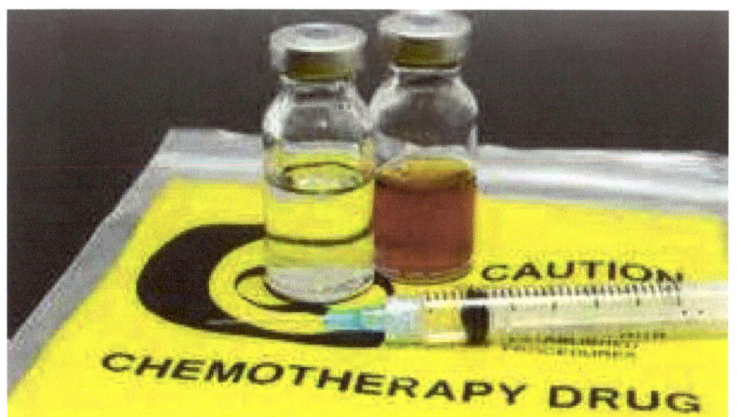

Chemotherapy for cancer is the use of medication to kill cancer cells. Contrary to radiation and surgery which are localized treatments, chemotherapy is a systemic treatment, which means that the medications travel throughout the whole body.

This means that the chemotherapy can reach cancer cells that may have spread or metastasized in other areas. Those of us who have had cancer, fear chemotherapy because of its violent and crushing effects on the human body, but we must accept that the essence of this breakthrough has saved many lives.

There are many opinions about it, but I will give it the benefit of the doubt because it cured me and it completely reduced my tumor. Therefore, I will make sure that this book lets you know some details about this method. I think it is worth it.

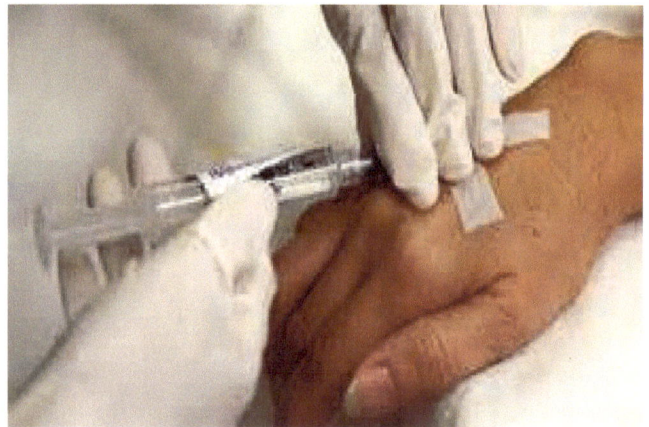

CHEMOTHERAPY IS USED IN FIVE DIFFERENT WAYS

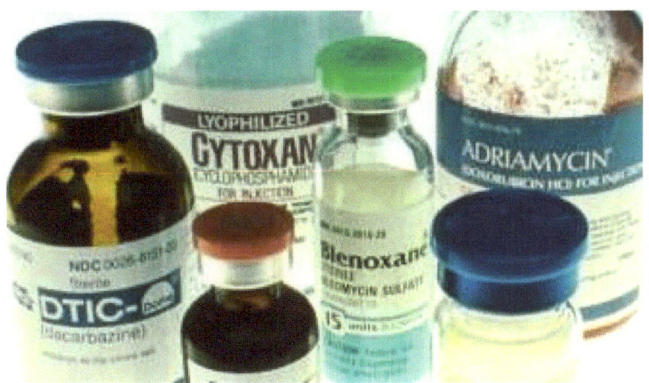

Adjuvant Therapy: Chemotherapy administered after surgery, either by itself or with radiation (or some other type of therapy) and which is designed to kill cells that might have spread.

Neoadjuvant chemotherapy: Chemotherapy used before surgery to shrink a tumor, usually administered along with radiotherapy. This is the one that I was given; eight treatments of chemotherapy.

Primary Therapy: This form is used alone in cases of leukemia or lymphoma. The therapy is also used alone to control other types of cancer when there is no hope for recovery and the chemotherapy is administered to control the symptoms.

Induction chemotherapy: Used as the first of many therapies. For instance, in treatments of some lung cancers, chemotherapy can be administered first by induction, followed by surgery or radiotherapy. In stomach cancers (before or after surgery) the chemotherapy can be administered first and followed by radiotherapy.

Combination chemotherapy: This chemo involves the use of two or more chemotherapeutic agents allowing each medication to increase the performance of the other so that the two may work synergically.

Normally the healthy cells submit to the cellular cycle in a regulated manner; while some cells are dividing and creating new cells, others are dying. Abnormal cells divide and reproduce uncontrollably, creating a mass of cells known as a tumor. Mine was 4 centimeters (1.5") big in the right breast.

The cellular cycle is important for chemotherapy since all chemotherapeutic medications are focused on and interrupt different phases of the cellular cycle. Most chemotherapeutic medications act upon reproducing cells. Since cancer cells actively reproduce, they are the primary focus of chemotherapeutic medications. This is what causes the side effects. When chemotherapy is administered, the doctor must find a balance between destroying the cancer cells and leaving the normal ones. This is why your hair falls out and your nails become weak. But what must be clearly understood, and which I consider to be very important in spite of all the side effects, is that chemotherapy has several objectives depending on the type of cancer that we may have.

Chemotherapy can cure: The objective is to cure cancer, so that it may disappear (to obliterate it) so that it may not return.

Chemotherapy can control: If a cure is not possible, the purpose of chemotherapy then is to control the growth and spread of cancer. And lastly, if a cure or control is not possible, chemotherapy is administered to alleviate the symptoms caused by cancer.

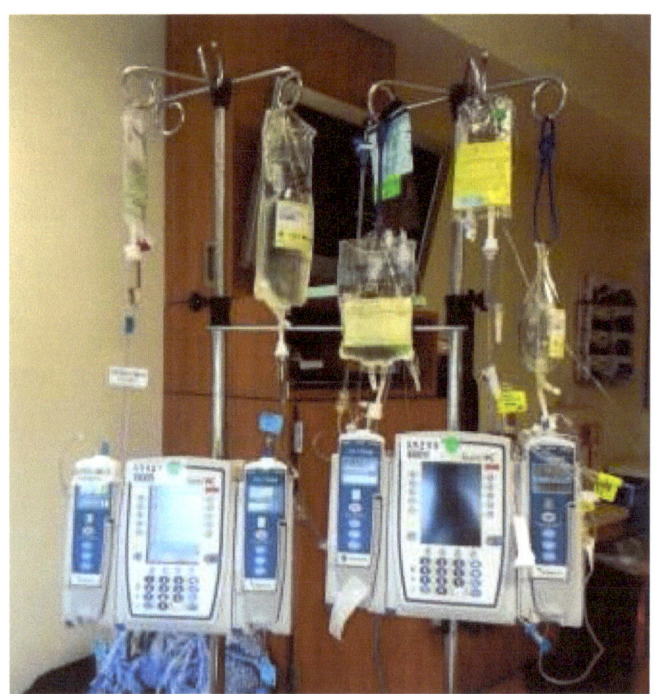

CHEMOTHERAPY USE, MY REJECTION, BUT AT THE SAME TIME, AWARENESS OF THE NEED

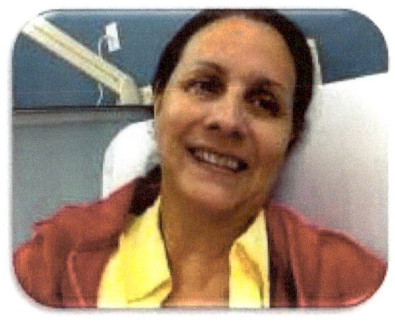

As an intelligent woman I am, I'm aware of the barbarity and ambiguity of the word chemotherapy. I feel the same as any person feels when he or she is on treatment, in fact, I have coped myself with eight chemotherapies *"We feel that we die during and after each treatment, but at the same time we feel that we can be saved from the disease."* It is an overwhelming cold that runs and weakens our bodies, and we know,

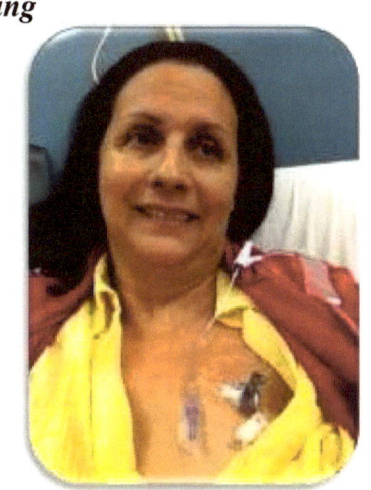

the most thoughtful ones, that the treatment is beating the cancer, but also, it is killing our good cells which give us life.

The chemotherapy is used to treat several types of cancer. The type, location, and phase of cancer, as well as your overall health, determine what kind of chemotherapy has to be applied and what factors should be used. For example, the adjuvant chemotherapy is considered as a standard treatment for the breast and colorectal cancer. The neo-adjuvant chemotherapy has been effectively used to treat breast cancer, bladder, esophagus, larynx and locally advanced non-small cell lung cancer.

The brain tumors are more difficult to treat with chemotherapy due to the protective effect of the blood–brain barrier, the tumor location within the skull, and the lack of an adequate lymphatic drainage. Because chemotherapy can kill healthy cells along with cancer cells, several side effects are associated with this type of treatment.

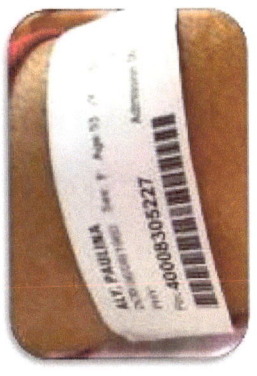The most common side effects occur in areas where the healthy cells are rapidly dividing. The blood cells, hair follicle cells, skin cells, cells of the reproductive and digestive tract.

That´s why I have said *"We feel that we die during and after each treatment, but at the same time we feel that we can be saved from the disease"* the side effects are strong.

The kind of side effects and how severe they are, will depend on the type and dose of chemotherapy and how your body reacts to it.

Some of the most common side effects are the fatigue, the hair loss, the lack of energy, the nausea and vomiting, because chemotherapy drugs irritate the stomach lining, and the first section of the small intestine (Duodenum) which stimulates certain nerves leading to the vomiting center of the brain.

This causes the nausea and vomiting. But also, we can do something to prevent when the nausea and vomiting persist. In my case, I used to drink liquids at least one hour before or after each meal, but never during the meal. I used to eat and drink slowly. It is something very important to eat several small meals throughout the day instead of larger ones; it is better for the stomach. Breathe deeply and strongly when you experience nausea. Avoid sweet, fried, oily or fatty foods. Take a break, but don't lie down until at least two hours after each meal. It is a difficult moment, but very necessary, therefore you should follow my advice about the food, because it works.

Also, drugs have been developed to help to control the nausea and vomiting associated with the chemotherapy, many of which can be extremely effective, I used to solve this problem with Lorazepam, Ondansetron, and on the worst day of the crisis with Dexamethasone (Dexamethasone, Hydrocortisone and Prednisone).

COMPLICATED PROCESS OF REFLECTION, OVERWHELMING BUT NECESSARY

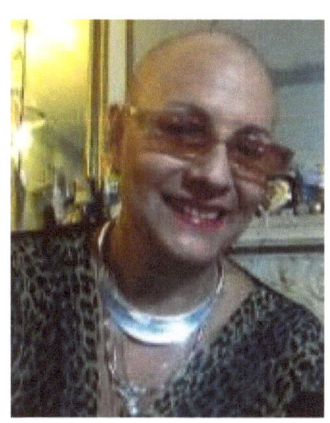

We spent the time trying that the others are better, being the supporting of many people, but, have you thought *how many of these people try that your life is better? How many of them are worried about what you feel?* It´s very complicated, but don´t get discouraged, the pace of life today has changed the parameters of the affectional behavior and all the generations that were brought up at an old fashionable way, started to stay in the past. There is a new global mechanism that manages the *social-carnal relations*, sometimes in an inconvenient way or incompatible with the principles we were educated with, but that is already irreversible.

In the past, the family was an indestructible maze, but today the changes that the societies are experiencing worldwide are in a large-scale transforming then the way of feeling, knowing and living. Children get away from parents, many women prefer to be single mothers and some others are obliged to, because the lack of love and the injustice for being abandoned by their love partners. In fact, the pattern where a father was the role model is disintegrating, and sometimes the tenderness in the families is disintegrating too, when they have to be separated to look for earning a living, it is here when the affective stuff disrupts and acquires other incredible nuances, but always keeping the distance and coldness, because the body cannot resist any more.

Imagine a person who has come to this country looking for a better future for his or her family, but as far as this person is achieving that supposed dream, it is found that the only option is being working for more than 15 hours or more, eat whatever is gotten, rest and go back to work next day, then wait for the payment to send money to the family left behind. That fatigues and involves the human being to an uncalculated stress that has to be overcome.

On the other hand, you have to be strong because:

- God is by your side in all your way of life
- Nobody is going to love you as you love yourself
- There are just few people who love us as we are in essence and this hurts a lot.
- The problem is ours, the others don´t have any obligation to afford it with us
- You cannot expect anything from others. Be self-sufficient.
- The pity is something terrible.

KNOWLEDGE OF THE CRUEL REALITY AROUND AS A LESSON

Today, I thank God for taking me off the blindfold from my eyes and for showing me the actual reality of the surrounding world. I could recognize everyone at once and definitely, and I could see their aura, and feel in many circumstances, the thought of people in front of me.

Sometimes the murmur of the other's thoughts is fearful. I have had and I have the divine grace for being able to listen and see the people's naked soul in some moments. It has been pretty bitter in some cases but sharply. **Revelations fulfilled with light.**

I feel joyfully fulfilled for that gift that the Creator has given to me and for so much life in return and because He lets me grow up with great purposes in this second opportunity. Neither the past time is important nor the ones who got apart before the fatigue of my pain. Today I understand them completely, but, if they were in this situation I wouldn´t behave that way.

I am concerned with the present, and I walk to an immediate future. Nothing else. I care about you who read this book today, I know it is very useful in order to realize where exactly your path takes you in difficult and unexpected moments. I care about sick people, who are abandoned occasionally by their children, by their mothers or spouses, they are important to me.

I am also concerned with the ones I mentioned at the beginning, the ones who abandoned me and who read these pages today and should learn from them ashamedly, I don´t reprimand these people, but I don´t forget their lack of love in my most difficult moments.

Disgracefully, **nobody** in this world is exempt of having cancer, the cancer doesn´t have a face, it can be manifested in anyone, as the one who goes to jail for crashing his or her car against somebody accidentally without being a murderer. He didn´t want to kill but he or she is guilty, and he or she must stay in prison some time. People who gets sick must comply with the treatment period dedicating all their strengths in order to overcome the situation and defeat the cancer.

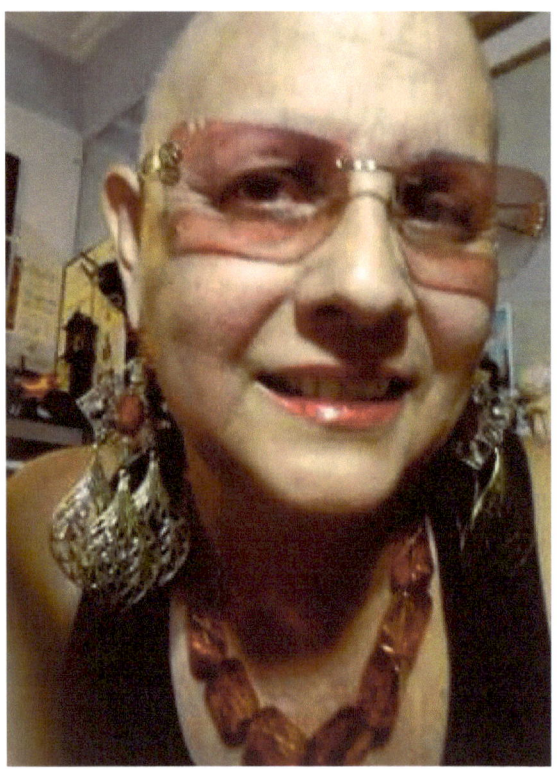

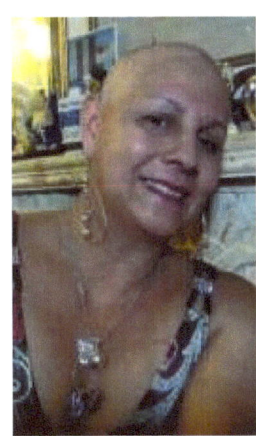
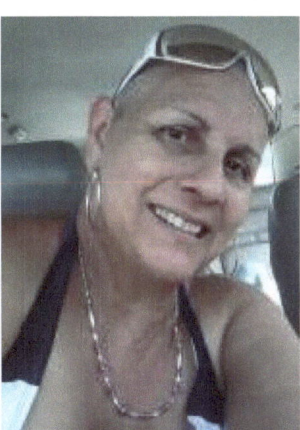
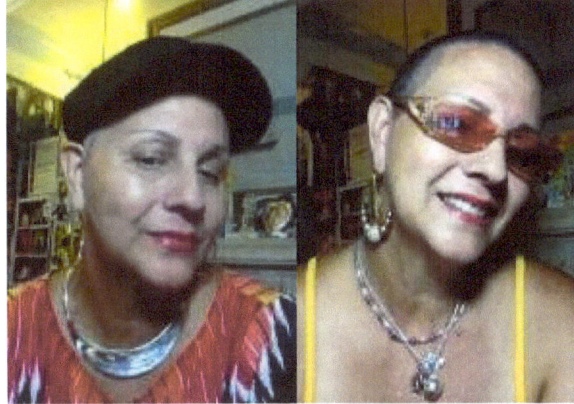

THE PAIN AFTER THE CHEMOTHERAPY IS CUMULATIVE

After the routine of one day of chemotherapy, more than seven days of pain come, also tiredness, sadness and a thousand of other things 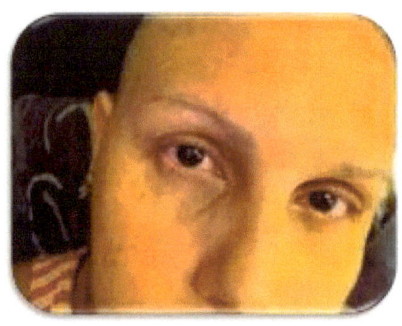 that only those who have experienced it, can understand when I say **THOUSANDS OF OTHER THINGS.**

Unfortunately, chemotherapy drugs can also cause painful side effects. These can damage nerves, more often in the fingers and toes, which lead to burning sensation, numbness, tingling or throbbing pain.

My nails first became gray, then black and some of them fell down, my ignorance on the subject took me by surprise and I had mouth ulcers too, but it was just at the beginning, because after reading and reading I discovered that if we put ice or ice-cream in our mouth on the first 45 minutes of treatment neither we will lose the sense of taste, nor will have ulcers. What do you think about it?

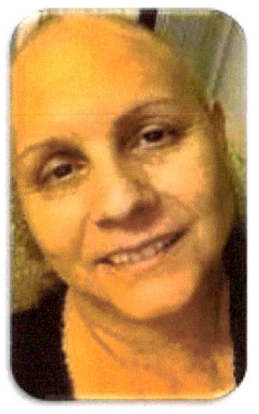

I was very affected by headaches and muscular pains, and also I could fight them with adequate medicines. To help your doctor determine how is the best way to control your pain, keep track of time, location, and characteristics of your pain and what you have done for getting better or worse. It is useful to develop a pain scale to describe how much pain you feel. Try to assign a number from 0 to 10; 0 means no pain at all and as your pain increases, so the number does too.

SICKNESS, DOUBTS, DEPRESSION AND FAITH

I recognize that I was acting in the same way as many people. As a weak person with insecurities, with fears that in my new me, nowadays have run away, today I am a warrior who enjoys every second from life.

I am convinced that with effort, kindness, joy, positivism, strictness and perseverance, all is possible. I also know that faith moves mountains.

Poor of those who live without faith!

Depending on the way we afford our problems, the sickness, the lacking of things and disillusions, according to the way we face them, the solution and the construction of our path will come anyway.

All can be achieved, it is just necessary a magical intention to go up by an honest and authentic way through our dreams.

For example, if you are diagnosed that you are really sick, I am going to use the word that many people don´t want to listen, *if you have CANCER*, the first I advise you is that you should assume you are sick. You should convince yourself that you can overcome it. It is not the end, remember that we are in this world just temporarily and for a short time, that´s why we should say:

> *We are going to beat it!*
>
> *We are still alive*
>
> *We have another second for living*

Think about the world, which is at least to me, made of the immediateness, of moments that we can accumulate second after second, and another and another until completing thousands of these seconds, which according to certain timers they become in minutes, hours, days and years…

I mean with all of this, that what it is worth is the present time, *what we do with our life, the second we can offer to humankind, starting with all of those who love, criticize and even hate us.* Remember that even those who hate us have loved us somehow in the past with a distorted feeling.

It is also that way if you have been abandoned, or if a loved one has passed away. You can overcome that moment of pain having faith in God and in yourself, being positive, letting away depressions, because depression only makes that the immunologic system decompensates and alters all the chemistry of our body, propitiating the emerging of infectious or cancerous diseases.

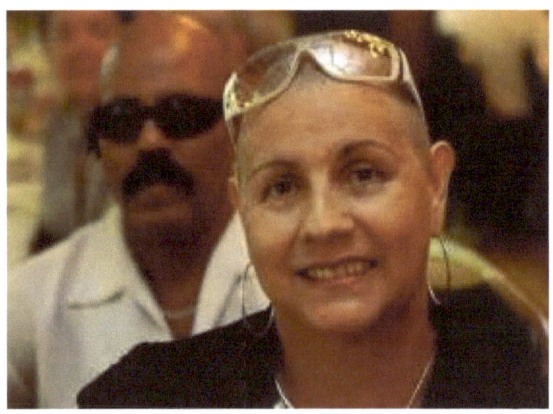

HAIR LOSS. A CHAPTER VERY IMPORTANT

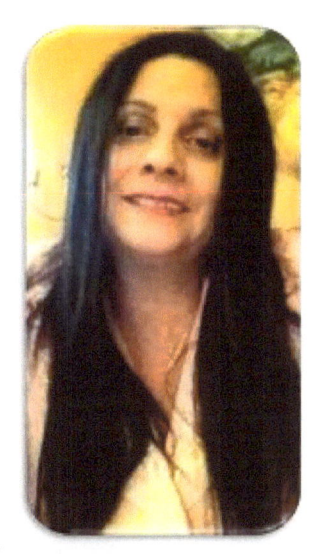

I want to emphasize this chapter of my life, because I think once the doctor determines the type of treatment, and the real possibility of losing their hair, people should cut it.

Why should they cut their hair? Well, I tell you with my hand on heart, the most acute and widespread pain that you can feel is the one when medicine attacks the follicles and then the hair falls, the medicine kills these cells and you pluck as a chicken.

Hair loss or alopecia, is a notable side effect of chemotherapy, but not all chemotherapy medications cause hair loss. Usually it occurs between 10 and 21 days after the drug administration. It could happen suddenly and with large amounts of hair or it could gradually fall. Hair loss is temporary and hair should grow back after treatment stops.

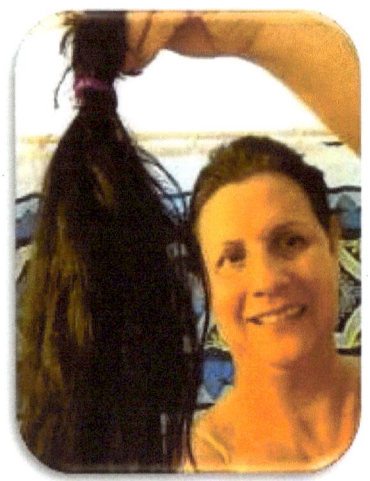

In my case, the day when I was told the kind of treatment I would receive and its consequences, I grabbed a scissors and cut all my hair, I shaved my head. It is also a healthy fact, because therapeutically speaking, hair is destined to fall gradually and this is something totally depressing.

In addition, you must become the master of the situation, don't let the cancer and the medicines manage your life. I have a Peruvian friend named **Guido Valdivia** who always told me *"Mrs. Paulina, the body is worth nothing, everything is in our mind"* and it is true, I've been able to transform my life by the commandment of my psyche, so I cut my hair, take a look at the mirror and said aloud, *"I have cancer and what? I will defeat it!"*

There were those who severely criticized me for uploading to social networks all photos of that day, but despite the adversity, despite the bad time I was living, I needed that everybody knew that I was fighting.

When you are able to leave the ego and shout out to the world *"I'm sick, but I'm going to fight for surviving"*, you survive for sure and this is my case, no matter what

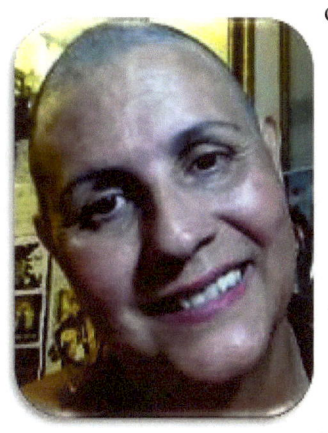

others think, because they are always going to think badly and talk badmouth of you, anyway, do not be naive.

Although it is not a life threatening, hair loss can be very annoying. Many people buy a wig or hairpiece, or use hats or scarves to cover their heads.

If you buy a wig because of cancer treatment, this is a tax-deductible expense and may be partly covered by your health insurance.

I tried to wear a wig one day because of the insistence of some people who I will not mention in this book. But I think it is inappropriate among so many symptoms, so many ailments, in the hot weather of Miami, wear a wig that squeezes your head.

I know that some snob ladies don't accept my ordinary way of thinking, but I'm so sorry, I take off my shirt to pain, to adverse situations and I don't care, but I advise you to be happy and free. Many women think that ***"their men"*** can leave them when they are hairless, but who can be interested in a man who thinks about the aesthetic aspect rather than the pain you are feeling, not only physical but mental, psychological. It is very strong when they tell you that ***"You have cancer"***.

WHEN I GOT ANEMIA, IT MEANS A LOW LEVEL OF RED BLOOD CELLS

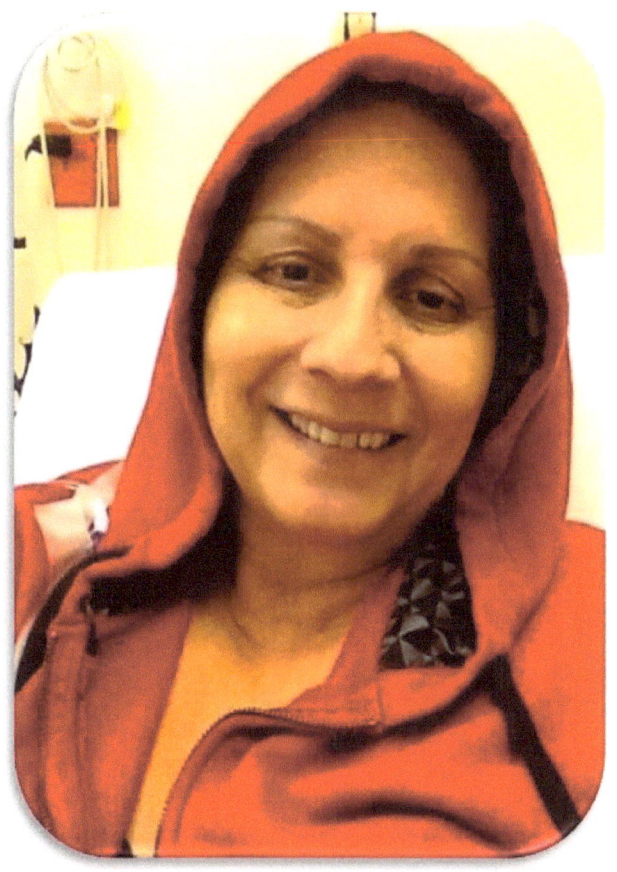

Every day I had to go to find out as I were an internet mouse, each detail that carried on my transformation through this bitter experience. **_THE CANCER_**.

My blood was suffering the decline of red blood cells, those cells that carry oxygen to all parts of my body. Finally, I knew why I was so tired, why I had dizziness, faintness and shortness of breath. Sometimes I felt that my heart is pounding or beating very fast, getting to have chest pain, but the worse could follow when I got nausea and vomiting.

Sometimes, we are not understood, it is pretended that we can get up and walk, but it is not possible. There are times when we can only obey the orders of our body and in my case, I rested a lot, slept or tried to sleep as much as I could at night and took several naps during the day.

I stopped doing many things that occupy every day of my life and I changed my diet, I started with a well-balanced diet. I learned that one may feel as if one were a thousand of years old. It hurts everywhere in my body, and as if I were an elderly woman I learned that I had to get up slowly. When I wanted to lay down I had first to sit down and then get up carefully.

Erythropoietin is a growth factor that occurs naturally which stimulates red blood cell production. Procrit and EPO are the types of the medicine. The drug was administered to me twice a week until the counting of the red blood cell increased.

LACK OF APPETITE AND THE IMMUNE SYSTEM

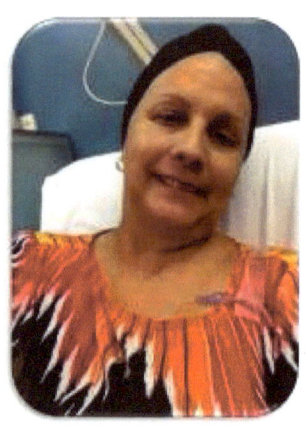

Many of chemotherapy drugs can cause a reduction or complete loss of appetite. Each person is different and there is no way to predict how the chemotherapy will affect you. But, loss of appetite and weight loss can vary from mild to severe and can lead to malnutrition.

Appetite reduction is usually temporary. Your appetite should return after the chemotherapy has stopped, but can last several weeks.

In my case it was tremendous, chemotherapy altered my sense of taste, the way how I taste and smell some food, but I didn't stop, I overcame everything and ate, appealed to my sense of reminder, my historical memory and thereby I could go forward. My weight remained, so I kept a little heavy.

In order to fight cancer and cope with chemotherapy, it is important for your body to get the proper nutrition. If you are experiencing loss of appetite, talk to your professional health care advisor; there are medications that can help. You cannot stop with it because if you develop malnutrition the chemotherapy effects can be almost fatal.

REMEDIES THAT WORKED TO KEEP FUNCTIONAL MY IMMUNE SYSTEM

Considering that the main function of the immune or defense system is to protect the organism from diseases caused by viruses, fungus, parasites and bacteria, I had to take very precise measurements when I was told I had an aggressive cancer.

The immune system fights against the harmful elements through lymphocytes (white blood cells) and antibodies (protein molecules)

All of this is supported by the lymphatic system, consisting of the spinal cord, the thymus, the lymph nodes, the spleen and the lymphoid tissue. However, sometimes, the immune system weakens leaving the body exposed to serious diseases. That was my case, too much work, very bad diet and a little of rest, all of this produced or increased the risk of getting cancer.

I had to search on my grandmother's books to find remedies to consolidate the immune system, because it was approaching a difficult stage of chemotherapies.

Among the popular remedies that I could adapt to my daily life, there were four which I took turns at the week strictly:

Remedy to consolidate the immune system number 1: Take one spoonful of honey daily on an empty stomach.

Remedy to consolidate the immune system number 2: Take a ginseng tea, which is known not only for preventing diseases, but also for the treatment of immune-related diseases, also on an empty stomach.

Remedy to consolidate the immune system number 3: Extract the juice of a regular sized carrot and two oranges and mix them. Take this mix daily at breakfast to stimulate the immune system.

Remedy to consolidate the immune system number 4: Pour 20 drops of dissolved propolis in some water and drink it three times a day. Propolis is a sort of natural resin made by bees; they cover the holes in the hive with it, preventing the spread of germs. It acts in our body as a bactericide, disinfectant and immune system enhancer.

Sometimes, it is not easy to consume certain remedies, but it is the only way we can be a little better.

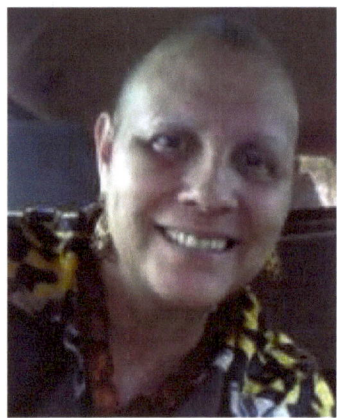

IF YOU EXPERIENCE MOUTH ULCERS TRY THE FOLLOWING TO HELP CONTROL THEM:

Ask your doctor to prescribe or recommend a medication to relieve pain; there are some remedies that could apply directly to the ulcers.

Consume cold foods at room temperature. Hot and warm foods can irritate a tender mouth and throat.

Eat soft and soothing foods, such as ice creams, milkshakes, baby food, soft fruits (bananas and apple puree), mashed potatoes, cooked cereals, boiled eggs or scrambled eggs, yogurt, cottage cheese, macaroni and cheese, and puddings.

Prepare puree in a blender with the cooked foods to make them softer and easier to eat.

Avoid irritants and acidic foods and juices, such as tomato juice and citrus; spicy or salty foods; and hard or rough foods such as raw vegetables, granola, popcorn, and toast bread.

If you are sick, follow these important advices to win the battle. Remember that the cancer can change the way the body utilize the food, and the cancer treatments can affect the nutrition.

- A diet of 80% of fresh vegetables and juices, grains, seeds, nuts, almonds and just some fruits lead the body to an alkaline environment. Only 20% can be consumed in cooked foods. Wash all fruits, vegetables and raw fresh herbs with normal and cold water to reduce the risk of infections.

- Fresh vegetables juices give the body coenzymes easy to absorb and get to the cells 15 minutes after its consumption for nurturing and helping the formation of healthy cells. To get live enzymes that help to build healthy cells, drink vegetables juices (almost all including alfalfa) and eat many fresh vegetables two or three times a day.

- The people with cancer often need more protein than usual. After surgery, the chemotherapy or radiotherapy normally it is needed additional protein to heal the tissues and help to defeat the infections. Among the good sources of protein are include red lean meat, eggs, dairy products, low fat, nuts, peanut butter, beans, peas, dry lentils and soy foods.

- The green tea is a better alternative and has properties that fight cancer.

- Eat frequently, a little each hour, don't wait until you are hungry.

- The water is better to drink purified or filtered to avoid toxins.

- Drink nutritious drinks high in calories like milkshakes and canned nutritional complements.

- Drink just pasteurized juices in cans or bottles.

- Because of cancer is also a disease of the mind, the body and the spirt, a more active and positive attitude will help the cancer patient to fight the disease and become a survivor.

- The anger and incomprehension, the non-forgiveness, stresses the body and put it in and acid ambience. Learning to have a kind and lovely spirit with a positive attitude is very beneficial for your health.

- Workout outdoors moderately.

- Take into account that some raw foods can contain microorganisms that can make a damage to your body when the cancer or treatment weakens your immune system.

- Be careful when you consume dairy products: All the milks, yogurt, cheese and other dairy products must have the pasteurized label in their containers.

- Eat neither soft cheeses nor blue streak ones (such as brie, camembert, Roquefort, stilton, gorgonzola and bleu). Don't eat Mexican style cheese such as fresh white and "cojita".

- Cook the food safely. When you cook make sure to use the proper time.

- Limit the number of very salty, smoked and marinated foods.

- Have to your disposal a variety of snacks rich in protein, easy to prepare and eat. For example, yogurt, cereal and milk, half of a sandwich, a plate nutritious soup, cheese and salty cookies.

- Learn to relax and enjoy life.

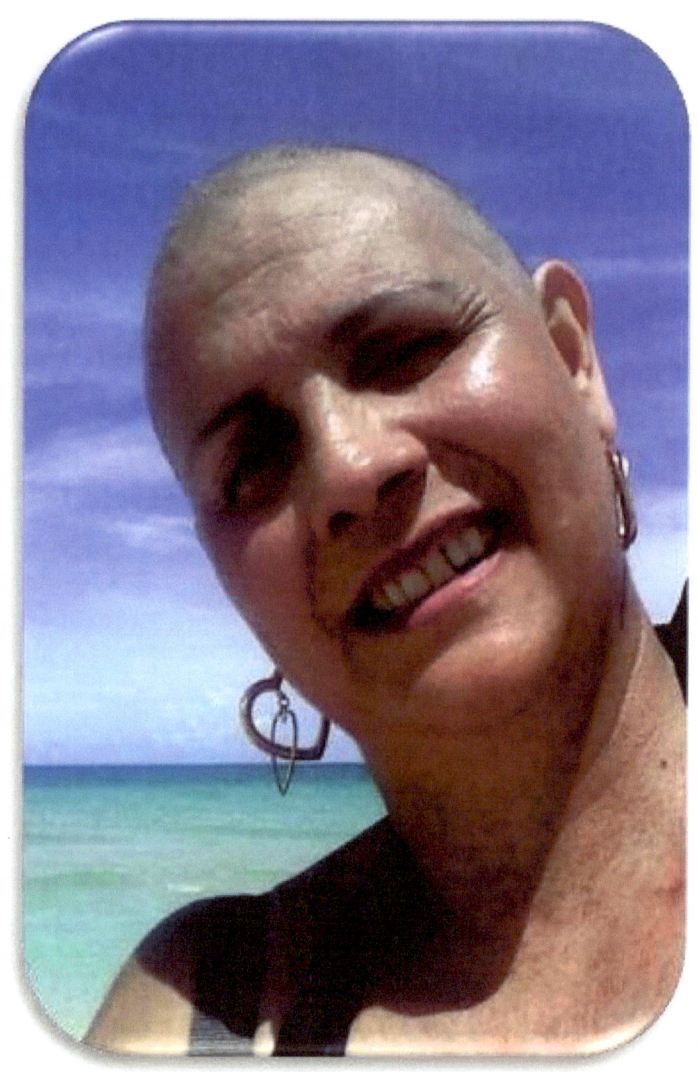

THE MOST EXPECTED DAY. MY SURGERY.

In spite of the fear that can be emerged when we know we are just about to enter to a surgery room, I can tell you that it was the most expected day out of the ten months of duration of my treatment. I was happy because of that November 22nd, 2013 had finally arrived.

The result from chemotherapies was wonderful, the tumor was completely reduced, and it means, my tumor disappeared, we have eradicated the carcinoma... What a joyful moment!

It was also a moment for important decisions:

1- **Who would be my surgeon?**

2- **Would I accept the surgery and just a quadrant were removed or would I sign for accepting a total mastectomy?**

3- **Would I authorize them for another procedure called Sentinel lymph node on that surgery date or not?**

Well, too many questions for a first time cancer patient, but always there is a first time in everything, and thanks God there is an effective and prolific Internet that help us to evaluate possibilities and know much better the scientific procedures worldwide today.

At the Jackson Memorial I had to wait for the operation in March until 2014, but in fact, I didn´t want to start a new year with the word Cancer in my life, and thus, I consulted my medical insurance and supported on Internet, I found Doctor **Adrian Legaspi,** an ordinary man but with a broad and excellent medical curriculum.

I found an appointment with this doctor quickly. That day he asked me *"when would you like to be operated?* "And I responded *"yesterday",* he smiled and told me that thanks to my medical analysis which were quite well it could be carried on by a week.

I considered that news extraordinary. We planned together about the surgery and about *"the Sentinel lymph node procedure"* which I have already checked out online and whose information seems very important to me, then I took notes about that in this book.

Doctor Legaspi agreed with me in everything, he would perform a total mastectomy and also the Sentinel lymph node procedure. Internet allowed me not to enter to the surgery and to the procedure without any knowledge of what they had to do on me. I saw about many radical mastectomies and about the lymph procedure.

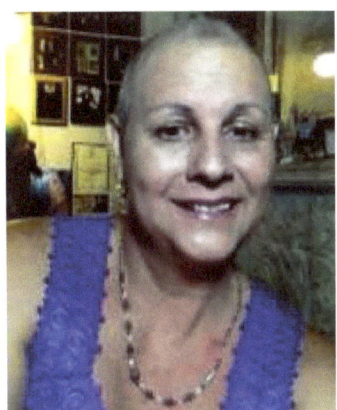

I was happy and convinced that it was the best and I was prepared for that day.

ENTRY TO THE MOUNT SINAI HOSPITAL. ALTON ROAD, MIAMI BEACH.

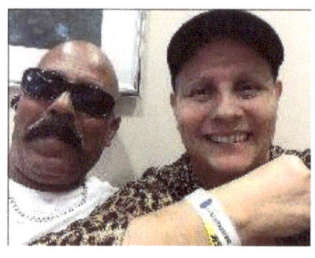

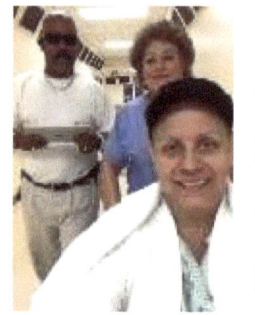

I came to the hospital ready to end the problem. After all documents were signed at the admission area, they took me to a small room where they will start with the Sentinel lymph node procedure.

The substance or colorant was injected before the surgery, I was quite happy because I would get out of this nightmare, also I was totally confident to Doctor Legaspi.

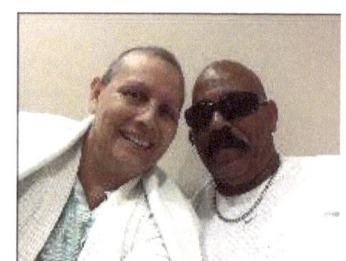

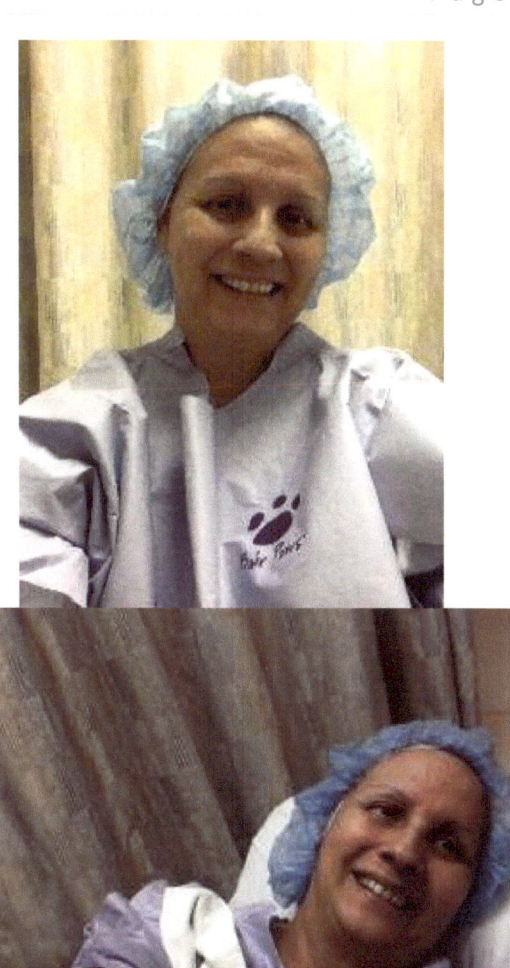

SENTINEL LYMPH NODE PROCEDURE

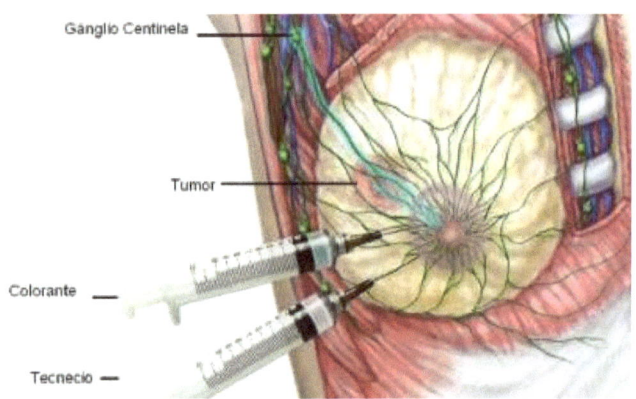

When I had to be faced to the continuous searching of information, I found with this procedure and talked to my doctor for performing this procedure to me.

When the cancer cells separate from the primary tumor (original) and go through the lymph or through blood until other parts of the body another tumor can be formed (secondary). This process is called metastasis. **The sentinel lymph node** is the first lymph node that the tumor cells find when they try to disseminate through the lymph. To identify the sentinel lymph nodes, a radioactive substance has to be injected, a blue ink or both in the subareoral area or near the tumor. The substance or ink goes through the lymphatic conducts until the lymph or the sentinel lymph node.

Next, it is used a system of detection (probe) to find the sentinel lymphatic nodes. Later, the surgeon only extracts the lymph nodes marked with the radioactive substance or the ink and a pathologist observe them at the microscope and determine if there are cancer cells or not.

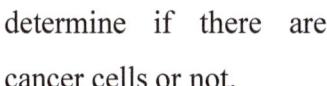

If the studio does not show malignant cells, the axillary dissection is not necessary. On the contrary, if it were positive, the axillary dissection should be done.

In my case it was positive, and thanks God, I had authorized this procedure and that Dr. Legaspi, a Hispanic doctor and an eminence on oncologic surgery, knew what he was doing.

Dr. Legaspi has offered me to do the quadrant surgery, because no tumor was anymore there, but I firmly said and we were convinced that a total mastectomy was the best, for avoiding risks and to be saved from radiotherapy after the surgery.

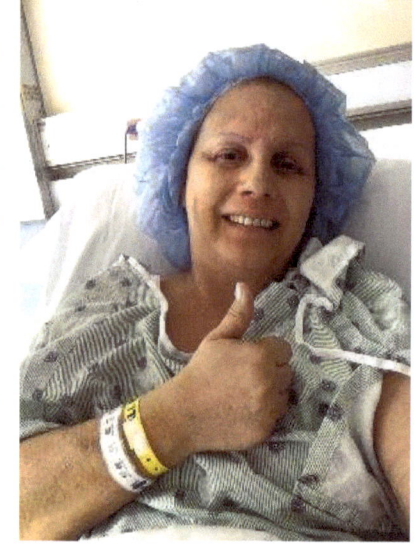

Effectively, when the sentinel lymph node procedure was made, 3 affected nodes were found, it means that they were marked with blue ink, when they were taken to pathology, microscopic cells with cancer remain in two of them. The nodes were extracted and an axillar dissection was made.

The detection and biopsy of the sentinel node, offers several conceptual advantages, comparing to the standard axillary dissection. The most remarkable for the patient is that it eliminates the risk of complications in a long term, avoiding the extensive axillary dissection, being the recovery process faster.

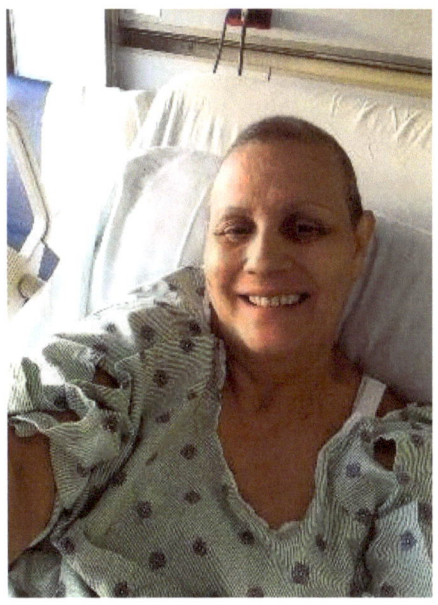

The surgery was a total success. There was a beautiful rainbow when I opened the curtain of the room, and it lasted just until I could see it and it was photographed by my husband.

REFLECTIONS FOR ANOTHER DECADE

When I talk to some of my friends much older than me, they told me *"but if you are a girl, you still have too much for living"* and when I hear that, I really think about it. If I have much more time for living, I have to reconsider how the next decade will be.

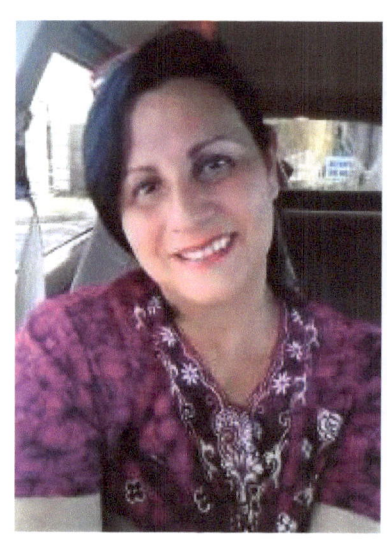

The communication with the ones who have lived more and gain us in advantages is important, because the perspective of life changes if I have another decade or if I have 30 years more for living, so my life should be totally different, it should be and must be better.

I remember my mother (R.I.P.) and it makes me feel sad, but I wouldn´t like to get older in the way he got. She died when she was 88. She was really deteriorated, asthmatic, in a sick-fat condition which stops her future.

On the other hand, there are people who spend their life pretending being who in fact they are not, they die if they don´t have an updated car, the best brand clothes, they really pretend acting in a way that is not correspondent to them and sometimes the funny thing is that they don´t have money not even for eating but they flaunt all these things. These people forget of other important details that have to be appreciated day after day in order to be able to go ahead through the path of our life.

In my case. I have lived my life trying and achieving endless dreams, goals, becoming words into teaching of life. Becoming my actions into firm resolutions, leaving a footstep where others can transit. I am proud of being this way.

It has been a difficult path, very difficult, full of thorns, full of stones, but also full of flowers and honey. I met loyalty and also met the overwhelming disloyalty, that one that slaps you in any afternoon without compassion. Nobody can told me a story about what life is, because I have been hungry, have been cold, have suffered the unloving, I have understood the actual sense of the existence.

Before I get sick I was so innocent, my face blushed easily. I could be trapped sometimes, but, at the end I also could overcome the problem or situation with a smile or with a teardrop. But, hey, this innocence didn´t get me far away from my deep thoughts and from my ideals, although I had to pay dearly along the years for it.

I can remember how my past has been, my first love, all those afternoons and nights, all those runaways, all those kisses and unforgettable moments of my youth years, how my childhood has been, how I was mocked in my teen years, how I suffered of bullying at the age of 15 which helped me to be where I am today.

I am able to close my eyes and cry as that day when I was very unhappy, when I was betrayed, when I was abandoned for the first time. Always that first time that cannot be forgotten, that cannot be taken out from the bottom of our hearts. When you are hurt by someone, that person doesn´t have any idea of the consequences that can be involved, especially when it was *"a first time* "for an innocent girl, with elderly parents, whose outings were only in a ´57 Plymouth car with her mother and father.

Then the definitive moment comes, where a wooden box contains that human being who gave your life, your father who will never forget and who died in your arms. It was terrible to see his face and his body lying down in that damaged coffin. I repeat, damaged coffin, being unable to do to anything and not to have more tears for crying and not to understand what was going on and what will happen tomorrow. Who will take you to school? Who will teach you how to take a bus? Who will help your mother to look for a job? Too many things, just at the age of 15.

Life ran quickly until I become the woman I am today, without complexities, having suffered another transformation at the age of 53, when I got sick of cancer.

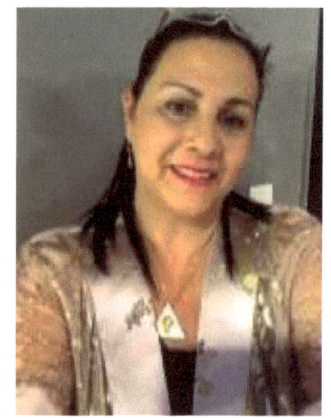

CHANGES AND REFLEXIONS

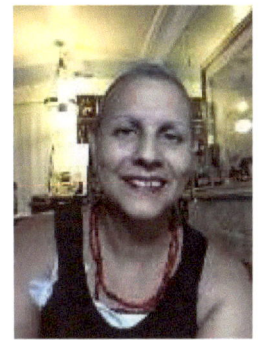

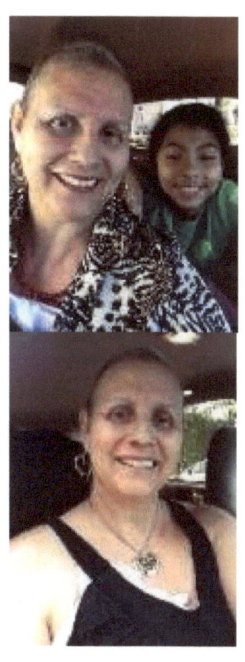

My life changed. It had to change. That´s why today, once I was cured of cancer, I started this campaign *"You will survive"* I need the world know what can be felt when you are in fullness youth and why it is necessary the prevention of diseases.

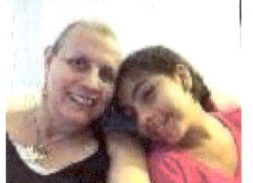

If my life changed, also your life can change positively.

Nothing is worth more than our families. That work that consumes us with the stress and is deteriorating our lives. The separations of family groups trying to get the *"American Dream"*.

People cannot be so resentful, you cannot live fighting all the time for money or for human miseries.

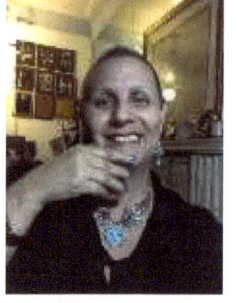

We should smile to life. All of us have the right of being instructed, to achieve the peace of our hearts. All of us have the right of SURVIVING, but not only of cancer, no, *we have to Survive* to the daily life, to the human discomfort, to the envy, to the badness. To the rich who look at you over your shoulder. To the miserable who is waiting for an opportunity of abusing you. To the heartless who hits a woman until she

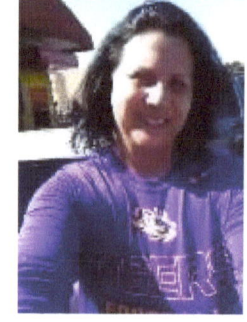

falls down. To whom is not able to coexist with a partner without mistreating. To whom doesn´t accept that a person loves another one of the same sex without being less person because of that. *All of us have the right to survive, not to be denied in our right to life and its pleasures given by the Lord. All of Us Have the Right to Survive to Our Own World Such as We Are.*

That´s enough about theories and supposed criterion of the how and what for Humankind was created. We have been created for giving historic continuity to a world which is almost ending and that will form, from its ashes another world then another one. We have contaminated our existence with perversity and egoism.

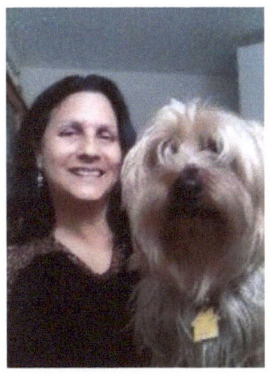

That is my conviction and that´s why I narrate my experience in this short book for those who haven´t suffered and can learn about a true experience on this subject, and for those who are suffering of cancer today or any other disease and can change the perception of their new life, which will never be as before. It will never be the same, I can ensure it.

Life changes us because our prism for observing it has now different nuances that we weren´t able to see before. That´s why the saying *"life depends on the prism you look at it"*.

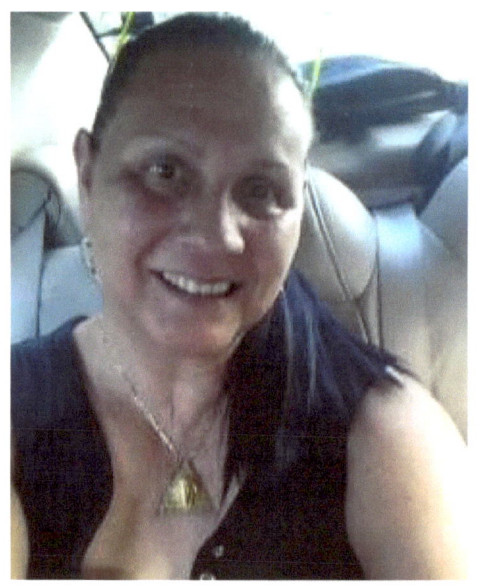

I thank God because I could grow up and get out of the shell where I lived, where the true was hidden by the innocence of my heart.

I am another woman. I have been born for the second time and only my GOD can detain me. Thanks to my family and friends for the support once again.

I love you.

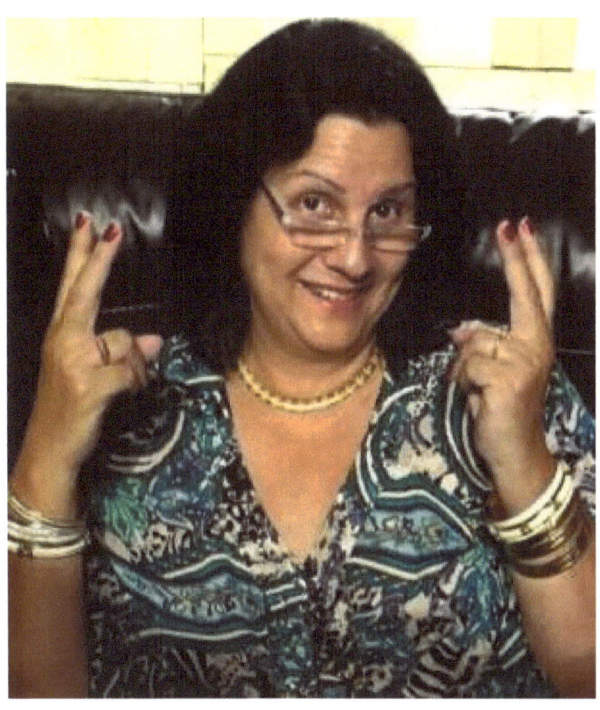

Certificate of the Importance of Life

I, _____ assume and accept the name that my parents gave me on the day _____ of the month of _____ the year _____.

I declare with my hand over my heart:

I am a child of God, unique and unrepeatable!

I declare that I am aware of all the responsibilities that He has entrusted me with, so that my world and that of my family is more enjoyable.

I agree to offer a smile to the rest of humanity.

I declare that I will place more attention to my mind so that it can reorganize the health of my body so that I will not consume unnecessary medicines.

That nobody will change the route of my winning spirit.

I declare that I am capable of winning over my illnesses with my positivity.

I declare that I am a winner in the name of our Lord all powerful and the Holy Spirit.

Signed_____

Date_____

Table of Contents

UNUSUAL DEDICATION 5

YOU WILL SURVIVE 9

GREATER KNOWLEDGE OF THE SUFFERING MAKES US HAVE ABSOLUTE CONTROL OF THE SITUATION 11

WHO IS PAULINA FATIMA? 14

NOTHING IS ETERNAL, NOT EVEN THE DEEPEST PAIN .. 18

MY 50 YEARS OLD. A GOOD STARTING POINT. 21

THE MOMENT OF TRUTH: THE FEAR 23

THE DEPRESSION AS STRONG AS THE CANCER 27

OVERCOME THE FEAR TO DEATH 29

CATHETER AND PORT DAY ON MY CHEST 35

CHEMOTHERAPY: A FATEFUL AND CONTROVERSIAL 37

CHEMOTHERAPY USE, MY REJECTION, BUT AT THE SAME TIME, AWARENESS OF THE NEED 43

COMPLICATED PROCESS OF REFLECTION, OVERWHELMING BUT NECESSARY 47

KNOWLEDGE OF THE CRUEL REALITY AROUND AS A LESSON 50

THE PAIN AFTER THE CHEMOTHERAPY IS CUMULATIVE 54

SICKNESS, DOUBTS, DEPRESSION AND FAITH 56

HAIR LOSS. A CHAPTER VERY IMPORTANT 59

WHEN I GOT ANEMIA, IT MEANS A LOW LEVEL OF RED BLOOD CELLS 63

LACK OF APPETITE AND THE IMMUNE SYSTEM 66

REMEDIES THAT WORKED TO KEEP FUNCTIONAL MY IMMUNE SYSTEM 68

IF YOU EXPERIENCE MOUTH ULCERS TRY THE FOLLOWING TO HELP CONTROL THEM: 71

THE MOST EXPECTED DAY. MY SURGERY. 77

ENTRY TO THE MOUNT SINAI HOSPITAL. ALTON ROAD, MIAMI BEACH. 80

REFLECTIONS FOR ANOTHER DECADE 86

CHANGES AND REFLEXIONS 91

www.ingramcontent.com/pod-product-compliance
Lightning Source LLC
Chambersburg PA
CBHW040826180526
45159CB00001B/85